BREATH OF HOPE:

CONQUERING TUBERCULOSIS FOR A BRIGHTER FUTURE

DR. MELISSA P. NELSON

TABLE OF CONTENTS

PREFACE

Welcome to "Breath of Hope: Conquering Tuberculosis for a Brighter Future, an exploration into the triumphs and tribulations of a battle that spans centuries. In these pages, you'll discover not only the scientific strides in defeating tuberculosis but also the stories of courage etched in the fight against this ancient adversary. As we embark on this journey, may the narratives within kindle a flame of optimism, and may the collective efforts showcased herein inspire a renewed commitment to a world where the breath of hope prevails over the shadows of disease. Your presence here signifies a shared commitment to a brighter, healthier future, where each breath is a testament to our resilience and unwavering spirit to conquer.

INTRODUCTION: THE SILENT THREAT

In the stillness of medical history, tuberculosis has emerged as a silent threat, weaving its tendrils through the fabric of societies across time. Unseen yet pervasive, it has claimed lives, altered destinies, and left an indelible mark on the collective human experience. As we delve into the pages of this book, we illuminate the shadows cast by this formidable adversary, setting the stage for a profound exploration into the importance of addressing tuberculosis in our quest for global health.

In focusing our lens on conquering tuberculosis, we embark on a journey that extends far beyond the laboratory and clinic. This is a narrative that unfolds through the resilience of individuals, the innovation of researchers, and the collective determination of communities. The tapestry we weave here is one of hope—a testament to our shared commitment to forging a brighter future, free from the shackles of this ancient ailment.

As we navigate through the chapters ahead, let us recognize tuberculosis not merely as a medical challenge but as a call to action. Through understanding, collaboration, and unwavering resolve, we aspire to transform the narrative surrounding this silent threat into a tale of triumph. Each word on these pages is an invitation to join hands in the pursuit of a world where the echo of every breath reverberates with the promise of health, resilience, and the dawn of a brighter tomorrow.

CHAPTER 1: UNDERSTANDING TUBERCULOSIS

Trying to solve the mystery that has endured throughout human history, we set out on a voyage into the complex world of TB in the first few pages of our investigation. Mycobacterium tuberculosis is the bacterium that causes tuberculosis, sometimes referred to as TB or TB in common language. Beyond its general character, TB presents in different ways, each of which poses particular difficulties for the individuals it affects and the medical professionals working to battle it. Each kind of TB, whether it affects the lungs directly or manifests extrapulmonary and targets other organs, requires our attention and comprehension.

Defining Tuberculosis and Its Different Forms

Tuberculosis (TB) is a potentially serious infectious disease caused by the bacterium Mycobacterium tuberculosis. This bacterium usually attacks the lungs but can also affect other parts of the body. TB is a global health concern, with millions of new cases reported each year. Understanding the different forms of tuberculosis is crucial for effective diagnosis, treatment, and prevention.

Forms of tuberculosis:

1. Pulmonary Tuberculosis (TB):

Overview: Pulmonary TB is the most common form and primarily affects the lungs.

Symptoms: Persistent cough, chest pain, coughing up blood, fatigue, weight loss, and night sweats.

Transmission: Airborne transmission through respiratory droplets occurs when an infected person coughs or sneezes.

2. Extrapulmonary Tuberculosis:

Overview: This form of TB affects parts of the body other than the lungs.

Examples: TB can impact the lymph nodes, bones, joints, central nervous system, and other organs.

Symptoms: Vary depending on the affected area and may include swelling, pain, or neurological symptoms.

3. Latent Tuberculosis Infection (LTBI):

Overview: In LTBI, the person carries the TB bacteria but does not show symptoms or feel sick. However, they can develop active TB later.

Diagnosis: Usually identified through a positive skin or blood test, without symptoms or signs of active disease.

Prevention: Treatment with antibiotics can prevent the progression of active TB.

4. Drug-Resistant Tuberculosis:

Overview: TB bacteria can develop resistance to the drugs commonly used to treat the infection.

Types: Multidrug-resistant TB (MDR TB) and extensively drug-resistant TB (XDR TB) are more challenging to treat.

Causes: Incomplete or improper treatment, which allows the bacteria to adapt and become resistant.

Diagnosis and Treatment:

- **Diagnostic Methods:**

Chest X-rays, sputum tests, and blood tests are common diagnostic tools.

Molecular tests, such as nucleic acid amplification tests, help identify the presence of TB bacteria more rapidly.

- **Treatment:**

Standard TB treatment involves a combination of antibiotics over a specified period, usually six to nine months.

Drug-resistant TB requires specialized and prolonged treatment regimens with second-line antibiotics.

Prevention:

- **Vaccination:**

Bacillus CalmetteGuérin (BCG) is a vaccine that can protect against severe forms of TB, especially in children.

- **Infection Control:**

Proper ventilation, isolation of infectious individuals, and the use of masks can help prevent TB transmission.

- **Treatment of Latent TB:**

Identifying and treating individuals with latent TB infection can prevent the development of active disease.

Tuberculosis remains a significant global health challenge, but with early diagnosis, appropriate treatment, and preventive measures, its impact can be mitigated. Understanding the different forms of tuberculosis is crucial for healthcare professionals to manage and control the spread of this infectious disease. Public health efforts, research, and international collaboration are essential in the ongoing fight against tuberculosis.

Providing an Overview of the Global Impact of TB

Tuberculosis (TB) is a global health concern that affects millions of people worldwide.
Here's an overview of the global impact of TB:

- **Prevalence:**

According to the World Health Organization (WHO), TB is one of the top 10 causes of death worldwide.

In 2020, an estimated 10 million people fell ill with TB, and around 1.5 million died from the disease.

TB is prevalent in both developed and developing countries, but the burden is higher in low and middle-income nations.

- **Transmission:**

TB is caused by the bacteria Mycobacterium tuberculosis, which primarily affects the lungs but can also target other parts of the body.

It spreads through the air when an infected person coughs or sneezes, releasing respiratory droplets containing the bacteria.

- **Social and Economic Impact:**

TB not only affects physical health but also has significant social and economic consequences.

The disease often strikes people in their most economically productive years, leading to a loss of productivity and income for individuals and families.

- **Vulnerable Populations:**

Certain populations are at higher risk, including those with compromised immune systems (e.g., HIV/AIDS patients), malnourished individuals, and people living in crowded or unsanitary conditions.

- **Global Distribution:**

While TB is present in all regions of the world, the burden is disproportionately high in certain areas, such as sub-Saharan Africa, Southeast Asia, and the Western Pacific.

India, China, Indonesia, the Philippines, Pakistan, and Nigeria are among the countries with the highest TB burdens.

- **Drug-resistant TB:**

The emergence of drug-resistant strains of TB, including multi-drug resistant TB (MDR TB) and extensively drug-resistant TB (XDR TB), poses a significant challenge.

Treating drug-resistant TB is more complex, lengthy, and expensive, making it harder to control.

- **Global Efforts:**

The WHO has implemented the End TB Strategy, aiming to reduce TB deaths by 95% and cut new cases by 90% between 2015 and 2035.

Efforts include improving diagnostics, expanding access to treatment, addressing social determinants of TB, and research into new drugs and vaccines.

- **Impact of COVID-19:**

The COVID-19 pandemic has disrupted TB services, leading to delays in diagnosis and treatment.

The focus on COVID-19 has diverted resources from TB programs, potentially exacerbating the TB burden.

- **Challenges:**

Challenges in the fight against TB include inadequate funding, stigma associated with the disease, limited access to healthcare, and the need for better diagnostic tools and treatment regimens.

- **Global Partnerships:**

International collaborations, such as the Global Fund to Fight AIDS, Tuberculosis, and Malaria, aim to mobilize resources and coordinate efforts to combat TB on a global scale.

Addressing the global impact of TB requires sustained efforts in prevention, diagnosis, and treatment, along with a focus on social determinants and the development of new tools and strategies. International cooperation and increased investment in TB programs are crucial for achieving significant progress in controlling and ultimately eliminating TB worldwide.

CHAPTER 2: HISTORICAL PERSPECTIVE

Tuberculosis (TB), one of the oldest diseases known to humanity, has left an indelible mark on history, shaping societies and influencing cultural perceptions. Examining the historical perspective of TB reveals a complex interplay between the disease, societal attitudes, and medical understanding.

Tracing the History of Tuberculosis and Its Societal Impact

The history of tuberculosis (TB) is a tale of humanity's struggle against a formidable adversary, a microbe that has left an indelible mark on societies across the ages. Tracing its roots reveals not only the medical dimensions of the disease but also its profound societal impact.

Early Encounters and Perceptions

TB has deep historical roots, with evidence suggesting its presence in ancient civilizations. Early descriptions resembling TB are found in texts from ancient Egypt and

India, revealing that the disease has been part of the human experience for millennia. In societies where medical understanding was limited, TB was often shrouded in mystery, with symptoms and outcomes attributed to supernatural forces or personal failings.

The Consumption Epidemic

As urbanization and industrialization took hold in the 18th and 19th centuries, TB became endemic, earning the ominous moniker "consumption." The crowded living conditions in burgeoning cities provided fertile ground for the spread of the disease. Entire families were often decimated, and communities lived in constant fear of its arrival. The impact was not merely physical; TB carried a significant societal burden, contributing to the creation of a culture of fear and stigma.

Sanatoriums and Isolation

With the understanding that TB was contagious, the 19th century saw the rise of sanatoriums as a response to the epidemic. These facilities, characterized by open spaces and exposure to fresh air and sunlight, aimed to isolate TB patients. While reflecting a proactive approach to disease control, this period also witnessed the stigmatization of those afflicted. Individuals with TB were often marginalized, and families faced ostracization from their communities.

A Bacterial Culprit and Diagnostic Advances

The late 19th century marked a turning point with the groundbreaking work of Robert Koch, who identified Mycobacterium tuberculosis as the bacterium responsible for TB. This discovery laid the foundation for diagnostic tools, including the tuberculin skin test. While advancing medical understanding, these developments also contributed to the identification and isolation of individuals with TB, intensifying the societal stigma associated with the disease.

Antibiotics and the Changing Narrative

The mid-20th century brought a transformative chapter with the discovery of antibiotics effective against TB. Streptomycin, isoniazid, and rifampicin turned TB from a nearly incurable disease into a curable one. This marked the beginning of the end of the pervasive fear surrounding TB. However, despite medical triumphs, societal challenges persisted as TB continued to disproportionately affect marginalized communities and individuals in poverty.

The Modern Era: Challenges and Progress

In the latter part of the 20th century, drug-resistant strains of TB emerged, posing new challenges. The HIV/AIDS epidemic further complicated the landscape, leading to a resurgence of TB in certain regions. Today, TB remains a global health concern with significant societal implications. The stigma persists, hindering efforts to diagnose and treat the disease effectively.

Tracing the history of tuberculosis is not just a journey through medical milestones but a narrative of human resilience and societal impact. From the fear-ridden days of consumption to the scientific breakthroughs of the antibiotic era, TB has left an enduring mark on societies worldwide. Understanding this history is essential as we navigate the contemporary landscape, striving to eliminate TB and mitigate its societal repercussions.

Advancements in Tuberculosis Research and Treatment

The battle against tuberculosis (TB) has witnessed remarkable strides in both research and treatment, ushering in a new era of hope and progress. In recent decades, concerted efforts from the global health community have led to significant breakthroughs that are reshaping our approach to TB.

- **Genomic Insights and Personalized Medicine:**

The advent of genomics has revolutionized our understanding of TB. Genome sequencing of Mycobacterium tuberculosis strains has provided valuable insights into the diversity of the bacterium and its adaptive strategies.

This genomic knowledge is crucial for developing personalized treatment regimens, taking into account the specific genetic makeup of the infecting strain. It contributes to more effective and tailored interventions.

- **Drug Development:**

Traditional TB treatment relied on a combination of antibiotics, such as isoniazid, rifampicin, ethambutol, and pyrazinamide. However, the emergence of drug-resistant strains necessitated the development of new drugs.

Bedaquiline and delamanid are examples of novel drugs approved for multidrug-resistant TB (MDR TB). Ongoing research focuses on expanding the arsenal of antiTB medications to combat resistant forms.

- **Vaccine Development:**

Bacillus Calmette-Guérin (BCG) has been the primary TB vaccine for decades, but its efficacy varies and it doesn't prevent adult pulmonary TB, the most common form of the disease.

Advancements in vaccine research include the development of candidates like M72/AS01E and RUTI. These vaccines aim to provide better protection against TB and may play a crucial role in preventive strategies.

- **Point of Care Diagnostics:**

Rapid and accurate diagnosis is essential for effective TB control. Traditional diagnostic methods, like sputum microscopy, have limitations.

Advances in molecular diagnostics, such as the GeneXpert system, allow for quicker and more accurate detection of TB and drug resistance. Point-of-care tests enhance accessibility, especially in resource-limited settings.

- **Immunotherapies:**

Immunotherapies represent a promising frontier in TB research. Approaches such as host-directed therapies aim to modulate the host immune response to enhance the body's ability to control TB infection.

Agents like interferons and immune checkpoint inhibitors are being explored to augment the immune response and improve treatment outcomes.

- **Digital Health and Data Analytics:**

Digital health technologies are playing an increasingly vital role in TB management. Mobile applications and telehealth platforms facilitate patient monitoring, medication adherence, and contact tracing.

Data analytics help in tracking disease trends, predicting outbreaks, and optimizing resource allocation for more effective public health interventions.

- **Global Collaborations and Funding Initiatives:**

Global partnerships, such as the Stop TB Partnership and the Global Fund to Fight AIDS, Tuberculosis, and Malaria, have played a crucial role in coordinating efforts and mobilizing resources.

Funding initiatives support research, drug development, and the implementation of comprehensive TB control programs globally.

- **Challenges and Future Directions:**

Despite these advancements, challenges remain. Access to new drugs and diagnostics in low-resource settings, addressing social determinants of TB, and combating stigma are ongoing priorities.

Continued research into host-pathogen interactions, identification of biomarkers for treatment response, and the development of shorter and more patient-friendly treatment regimens are key areas for future exploration.

In the dynamic landscape of TB research and treatment, collaboration, innovation, and a commitment to equity are driving forces. The ongoing efforts of researchers, healthcare professionals, and global health organizations give hope that a TB-free world is an achievable goal.

CHAPTER 3: THE GLOBAL BURDEN OF TUBERCULOSIS

Tuberculosis (TB) continues to be a major global health concern, affecting millions of individuals and communities worldwide. This chapter delves into the prevalence of TB across different regions, highlighting challenges and disparities in TB healthcare

Analyzing the Prevalence of Tuberculosis in Different Regions

Understanding the global distribution of tuberculosis (TB) is essential for developing effective public health strategies. This analysis explores the prevalence of TB in various regions, shedding light on the complex factors that contribute to its incidence.

- ### SubSaharan Africa: A Pervasive Challenge

SubSaharan Africa bears a significant burden of TB, with a high prevalence of the disease. Several factors contribute to this situation, including:

HIV/AIDS Epidemic: The co-epidemic of TB and HIV/AIDS is a major driver of TB prevalence in this region. HIV weakens the immune system, making individuals more susceptible to TB infection.

Socioeconomic Factors: Poverty, malnutrition, and limited access to healthcare services contribute to the persistence of TB. Crowded living conditions in urban areas facilitate the spread of the disease.

- **Southeast Asia: Densely Populated Hotspots**

Countries in Southeast Asia, such as India and Indonesia, face substantial challenges in controlling TB due to:

Population Density: Dense populations in urban areas create favorable conditions for the transmission of TB. Overcrowded living spaces and limited resources contribute to the challenges.

Healthcare Infrastructure: Uneven healthcare infrastructure and limited access to quality healthcare services hinder early diagnosis and effective treatment.

- **Western Pacific: Urbanization and Varied Challenges**

The Western Pacific region, including countries like China and the Philippines, grapples with diverse challenges related to TB:

Urbanization: Rapid urbanization leads to crowded living conditions, facilitating the transmission of TB. Urban areas often struggle with providing adequate healthcare services.

Healthcare Infrastructure: Disparities in healthcare infrastructure and access contribute to variations in TB prevalence within the region.

- **Eastern Europe and Central Asia: Transition Challenges**

This region has made progress, but challenges persist due to:

Drug-Resistant TB: Some countries in this region face challenges associated with drug-resistant TB, requiring specialized treatments and healthcare system adaptations.

Health System Restructuring: Post-Soviet era health system restructuring has presented obstacles to TB control efforts.

- **Latin America: Socioeconomic Determinants**

Latin American countries experience variations in TB prevalence influenced by:

Social Determinants: Socioeconomic factors, including poverty and inequality, contribute to TB incidence. Vulnerable populations face challenges in accessing healthcare.

Urbanization: Rapid urbanization and informal settlements create conditions conducive to TB transmission.

- **Middle East: Conflict and Displacement**

TB prevalence in the Middle East is influenced by unique factors:

Conflict and Displacement: Regions affected by conflict and large-scale displacement face challenges in maintaining effective healthcare services, leading to an increased burden of TB.

Varied Healthcare Infrastructures: Disparities in healthcare infrastructure among countries in the Middle East contribute to variations in TB prevalence.

- **Global Initiatives for Addressing Regional Disparities**

Global initiatives, such as the End TB Strategy led by the World Health Organization, aim to address these regional disparities by:

Strengthening Health Systems: Improving healthcare infrastructure and strengthening health systems to enhance early diagnosis and treatment.

Addressing Social Determinants: Recognizing and addressing social determinants, including poverty and inequality, to reduce vulnerability to TB.

International Collaborations: Fostering international collaborations and partnerships to mobilize resources and share best practices for TB control.

As we analyze TB prevalence across different regions, it becomes evident that a multifaceted and region-specific approach is essential. Tailored interventions, coupled with global collaboration, are vital in the ongoing efforts to reduce the global burden of tuberculosis.

Discussing Challenges and Disparities in TB Healthcare

Tuberculosis (TB) healthcare faces multifaceted challenges and disparities, hindering efforts to control and eliminate the disease. This discussion explores the key issues that contribute to these challenges and highlights the disparities in TB healthcare globally.

Socioeconomic Disparities:

- **Poverty and Limited Access:**

Challenge: TB and poverty share a symbiotic relationship. Impoverished individuals often face challenges in accessing healthcare services, leading to delayed diagnosis and treatment initiation.

Impact: Limited resources and inadequate healthcare infrastructure contribute to the persistence of TB in economically disadvantaged communities.

Access to Diagnosis and Treatment:

- **Diagnostic Challenges:**

Challenge: In many regions, especially low-resource settings, access to accurate and timely diagnostics remains a significant hurdle. Traditional methods may be the primary means of diagnosis, leading to delayed detection.

Impact: Delayed diagnosis not only affects individual patient outcomes but also contributes to the ongoing transmission of the disease within communities.

- **Treatment Gaps:**

Challenge: Despite the availability of effective treatments, gaps exist in ensuring universal access to them. This is particularly evident in regions with weak healthcare infrastructures.

Impact: Drug-resistant TB strains further complicate treatment regimens, requiring specialized medications and prolonged treatment plans, which are often challenging to implement.

Social Determinants:

- **Stigma:**

Challenge: Stigmatization of TB patients persists globally, impeding individuals from seeking timely medical attention. Fear of social isolation and discrimination discourages the disclosure of TB status.

Impact: Stigma contributes to delayed diagnosis, treatment abandonment, and the perpetuation of myths and misconceptions surrounding the disease.

- **Migration and Urbanization:**

Challenge: Movement of populations, whether due to migration or rapid urbanization, contributes to the spread of TB. Urban areas with dense populations and inadequate living conditions become hotspots for the disease.

Impact: The dynamics of migration and urbanization create challenges in tracking and treating TB cases, particularly in transient populations.

Coinfections and Vulnerable Populations:

- **HIV/AIDS Coinfection:**

Challenge: The intersection of TB and HIV/AIDS presents a significant challenge. HIV weakens the immune system, making individuals more susceptible to TB and complicating treatment strategies.

Impact: The co-infection increases the severity of both diseases and requires integrated healthcare approaches to manage these complex cases effectively.

- **Vulnerable Groups:**

Challenge: Disparities are observed among vulnerable populations, including refugees, prisoners, and those living in informal settlements. Limited access to healthcare exacerbates the impact of TB on these groups.

Impact: The vulnerability of these populations amplifies the challenges of TB control, requiring targeted and culturally sensitive interventions.

Disparities in Global Regions:

- **Regional Variations:**

Challenge: TB prevalence and control efforts vary significantly across regions. Factors such as socioeconomic conditions, healthcare infrastructure, and regional conflicts contribute to these disparities.

Impact: The variations highlight the need for tailored interventions and targeted resource allocation to address the specific challenges faced by different regions.

Global Initiatives and Future Directions:

- ### The End-TB Strategy:

Initiative: The World Health Organization's End TB Strategy aims to address disparities by emphasizing integrated, patient-centered care, prevention, and addressing social determinants.

Impact: Implementing comprehensive strategies that focus on both medical and social aspects is crucial for reducing disparities and improving overall TB healthcare outcomes.

- ### Global Collaborations:

Initiative: Collaborative efforts, including international partnerships and funding initiatives, play a pivotal role in mobilizing resources and sharing best practices.

Impact: Global collaborations contribute to research, innovation, and the implementation of effective TB control programs, fostering a more coordinated and impactful response.

In conclusion, addressing challenges and disparities in TB healthcare requires a holistic approach. Efforts must extend beyond medical interventions to encompass social determinants, economic disparities, and global collaborations. Achieving equitable access to high-quality TB healthcare is an ongoing challenge but is essential for realizing the vision of a world free from the burden of tuberculosis.

CHAPTER 4: TB DIAGNOSIS AND TREATMENT

Tuberculosis (TB) diagnosis and treatment are critical components in the global effort to control and eliminate this infectious disease. This chapter provides insights into various methods of diagnosing TB and outlines the treatment options available.

Methods for Diagnosing Tuberculosis

Accurate and timely diagnosis is crucial for the effective management and control of tuberculosis (TB). Various methods are employed to diagnose TB, ranging from traditional techniques to advanced molecular diagnostics. Understanding and utilizing these methods are essential for early detection and appropriate intervention.

Here are some key methods for diagnosing tuberculosis:

- **Tuberculin Skin Test (TST):**

Method: A small amount of purified protein derivative (PPD) tuberculin is injected just beneath the skin.

Principle: Measures the delayed hypersensitivity reaction to TB antigens.

Use: Primarily used for screening and assessing latent TB infection.

- **Interferon-Gamma Release Assays (IGRAs):**

Method: Blood tests that measure the release of interferon-gamma in response to TB-specific antigens.

Principle: Detects immune response to TB infection.

Use: Similar to TST, IGRAs are used for detecting latent TB infection, particularly in populations vaccinated with Bacillus Calmette-Guérin (BCG).

- **Chest X-ray:**

Method: Imaging of the chest to visualize abnormalities such as lung lesions, cavities, or infiltrates.

Principle: Identification of pulmonary abnormalities associated with active TB.

Use: Essential for diagnosing active pulmonary TB and assessing disease severity.

- **Sputum Microscopy:**

Method: Microscopic examination of sputum samples for the presence of acid-fast bacilli (AFB).

Principle: Detection of TB bacilli in respiratory secretions.

Use: Widely used for diagnosing pulmonary TB, but it has limitations in sensitivity, especially in HIV coinfection.

- **Molecular Tests (e.g., GeneXpert):**

Method: Detects the genetic material of Mycobacterium tuberculosis using molecular techniques.

Principle: Rapid and accurate identification of TB DNA.

Use: Highly effective in diagnosing TB, including drug-resistant strains. GeneXpert is a widely used molecular diagnostic tool.

- **Culture and Drug Sensitivity Testing:**

Method: Culturing the bacteria from a clinical specimen and testing its sensitivity to various drugs.

Principle: Identifying the specific strain of Mycobacterium tuberculosis and determining drug resistance.

Use: Essential for confirming TB diagnosis and identifying drug-resistant strains.

- **Bronchoscopy and Bronchoalveolar Lavage (BAL):**

Method: A bronchoscope is used to examine the airways, and BAL is performed to collect fluid for analysis.

Principle: Direct visualization and collection of samples from the lungs.

Use: Useful in obtaining specimens for culture when sputum samples are challenging to obtain.

- **Serological Tests:**

Method: Blood tests that detect antibodies against TB.

Principle: Measurement of the immune response to TB infection.

Use: Controversial due to variable accuracy and inability to differentiate between latent and active infection; not recommended for routine diagnosis.

- **Biopsy and Histopathology:**

Method: Tissue biopsy, often from lymph nodes or other affected areas, followed by histopathological examination.

Principle: Identification of TB granulomas or other characteristic tissue changes.

Use: Useful in extrapulmonary TB cases or when other diagnostic methods are inconclusive.

- **Point of Care Tests:**

Method: Rapid diagnostic tests performed near the patient.

Principle: Quick and onsite detection of TB or drug resistance.

Use: Improves access to diagnostics, especially in resource-limited settings.

Each diagnostic method has its strengths and limitations, and the choice of method often depends on factors such as clinical presentation, available resources, and the prevalence of drug-resistant TB in a particular region. In practice, a combination of these methods is often employed to achieve the most accurate diagnosis and guide appropriate treatment.

Various Treatment Options and Their Effectiveness in Tuberculosis

Effectively treating tuberculosis (TB) involves a combination of antimicrobial drugs, and the choice of treatment depends on factors such as the type of TB (pulmonary or extrapulmonary), drug susceptibility, and patient-specific considerations. Here, we detail various treatment options and their effectiveness:

- **First-line Anti-TB Drugs:**

Overview: The cornerstone of TB treatment involves a standard combination of four first-line drugs.

Drugs:

Isoniazid (INH)

Rifampicin (RIF)

Ethambutol (EMB)

Pyrazinamide (PZA)

Effectiveness: Highly effective against drug-susceptible TB when taken consistently.

- **Directly Observed Therapy (DOT):**

Overview: A strategy where a healthcare worker observes the patient taking their antiTB medications.

Effectiveness: Enhances treatment adherence, crucial for preventing drug resistance.

- **Drug-resistant TB Treatment:**

Overview: Drug-resistant TB requires different regimens, often involving second-line drugs.

Drugs:

Fluoroquinolones (e.g., levofloxacin, moxifloxacin)

Injectable drugs (e.g., amikacin, kanamycin)

Second-line oral drugs (e.g., ethionamide, linezolid)

Effectiveness: Success rates are lower compared to drug-susceptible TB, and treatment duration can extend to 20 months or more.

- **Fixed Dose Combinations (FDCs):**

Overview: FDCs combine multiple antiTB drugs into a single tablet, simplifying treatment.

Effectiveness: Improves adherence and reduces the risk of improper drug intake.

- **Treatment of Latent TB Infection:**

Overview: Individuals with latent TB infection may receive preventive therapy to reduce the risk of developing active TB.

Drugs: Isoniazid (INH) is commonly used for preventive therapy.

Effectiveness: reduces the progression to active disease and prevents transmission.

- **Vaccination (BCG):**

Overview: Bacillus Calmette-Guérin (BCG) vaccine is used in some regions to prevent severe forms of childhood TB.

Effectiveness: Provides variable protection against severe forms of TB, but its efficacy against pulmonary TB in adults is limited.

- **Shorter Treatment Regimens:**

Research Focus: Ongoing efforts to develop shorter and more patient-friendly treatment regimens.

Potential Impact: Improving adherence and reducing the burden on healthcare systems.

- **New Drug Development:**

Research Focus: Ongoing research into novel antiTB drugs.

Potential Impact: Addressing drug-resistant strains and improving treatment outcomes.

- **Vaccine Research:**

Research Focus: Developing more effective TB vaccines.

Potential Impact: Enhancing preventive strategies and reducing the global burden of TB.

- **Individualized Treatment Plans:**

Overview: Tailoring treatment based on patient factors, drug susceptibility, and comorbidities.

Effectiveness: Individualized plans optimize treatment outcomes by considering specific patient needs.

- **Adherence Support Programs:**

Overview: Educational programs, counseling, and support to ensure patients adhere to the prescribed treatment.

Effectiveness: Critical for the success of TB treatment, especially in long-term regimens.

Global Collaborations and Funding Initiatives:

Overview: International efforts to provide resources and support for TB treatment programs.

Effectiveness: Mobilizes funds for research, drug development, and healthcare infrastructure improvement.

- **Patient Monitoring and Follow-Up:**

Overview: Regular monitoring of treatment response through clinical and laboratory assessments.

Effectiveness: Ensures early detection of treatment failure or adverse effects, allowing timely adjustments.

- **Innovative Diagnostic Technologies:**

Overview: Adoption of advanced diagnostic tools like GeneXpert for rapid and accurate diagnosis.

Effectiveness: Facilitates prompt initiation of appropriate treatment.

While advancements have been made in TB treatment, challenges persist, particularly in the context of drug-resistant strains and treatment adherence. Continuous research, innovation, and international collaboration are vital for improving treatment options, ensuring global access to effective therapies, and ultimately achieving the goal of a TB-free world.

CHAPTER 5: LIVING WITH TB

Living with tuberculosis (TB) is a journey marked by challenges, resilience, and the profound impact the disease has on individuals and their communities. In this exploration of life with TB, we delve into personal stories, the social dimensions, and the emotional toll that TB imparts.

Sharing Personal Stories of Resilience: Living with Tuberculosis

In the shadows of a tuberculosis (TB) diagnosis, personal stories emerge—tales of resilience, courage, and the transformative power of community. Here, we share the narratives of individuals whose lives have been touched by TB, illuminating the human side of the disease.

1. Maria's Journey: Breaking the Chains of Stigma

Maria, a 32-year-old residing in a small rural community, found herself facing not only the physical challenges of TB but also the insidious stigma that surrounded the disease.

Determined to break the chains of silence, Maria decided to share her journey openly with her community.

In recounting her experiences, Maria highlighted the initial fear and misconception that surrounded her diagnosis. Friends and neighbors, driven by ignorance, distanced themselves. However, Maria's courage and willingness to educate her community gradually chipped away at the walls of stigma. She became a beacon of hope and information, inspiring others to seek an early diagnosis and adhere to treatment.

Maria's story emphasizes the transformative power of personal narratives in dispelling myths and fostering understanding within communities. Through her advocacy, she turned the tide from fear to compassion, paving the way for others to confront TB without shame.

2. Raj's Battle: Navigating the Complexities of Drug-Resistant TB

Raj, a vibrant young professional, found himself thrust into the complex world of drug-resistant TB. His journey was marked by challenges that extended beyond the physical toll of the disease. The long and arduous treatment regimen, coupled with the side effects of potent medications, tested Raj's resilience.

What emerged from Raj's story was not just a chronicle of medical treatments but a testament to the importance of comprehensive support systems. His battle against drug-resistant TB required not only medical intervention but also emotional and psychological support. Raj's experience underscores the need for holistic care that recognizes the multifaceted impact of TB on individuals.

Raj's narrative serves as a reminder that living with TB is not merely a medical struggle—it is a journey that demands understanding, empathy, and a community that stands as a pillar of support.

A Tapestry of Resilience: Beyond Diagnosis

These personal stories, interwoven into the broader tapestry of TB experiences, reveal common threads of resilience, community, and the need for a holistic approach to healthcare. They underscore the importance of sharing personal narratives to reduce stigma, increase awareness, and foster empathy within societies.

Beyond the diagnosis lies a rich narrative of individuals who, despite the challenges, have emerged stronger and more determined to contribute to the broader conversation on TB. Their stories serve as a call to action, urging communities, healthcare providers, and policymakers to approach TB not only as a medical condition but as a shared human experience.

In the collective sharing of these stories, a powerful narrative emerges—one that transcends borders and resonates with individuals globally. It is a narrative that invites us to listen, learn, and stand in solidarity with those living with TB, fostering a world where compassion and understanding prevail over stigma and fear.

Addressing the Social and Emotional Aspects of Tuberculosis

Tuberculosis (TB) not only affects the body but also leaves a profound impact on the social and emotional well-being of individuals. Addressing these aspects is essential for comprehensive care and to reduce the stigma associated with the disease.

- **Stigma and Discrimination:**

Challenges: TB is often shrouded in stigma, leading to discrimination and isolation of those affected. Fear of rejection may hinder individuals from seeking timely care.

Addressing Stigma:
Community Education: Launching communitywide education programs to dispel myths and misconceptions about TB.
Personal Stories: Sharing personal narratives of individuals who have overcome TB to humanize the experience.

- **The Impact on Mental Health:**

Challenges: The emotional toll of TB can lead to anxiety, depression, and fear, affecting both individuals and their families.

Mental Health Support:
Integrated Care: Incorporating mental health services into TB care for a holistic approach.
Counseling: Providing counseling services to help individuals cope with the emotional challenges of living with TB.

- **Family and Community Dynamics:**

Challenges: TB disrupts family and community dynamics, leading to economic strain, emotional distress, and social isolation.

CommunityBased Interventions:
 Support Groups: Establishing community support groups to create networks of understanding.
 Education Programs: Implementing programs that educate families and communities about TB to reduce fear and isolation.

- **Coping Strategies and Support Systems:**

Challenges: Individuals with TB need robust support systems to cope with the challenges of the disease.

Support Initiatives:
 Peer Support Groups: Creating spaces for individuals to share experiences, offer support, and provide practical advice.
 Educational Campaigns: Conducting campaigns in workplaces and schools to build understanding and empathy.

- **The Role of Healthcare Providers:**

Challenges: Healthcare providers must not only treat the physical symptoms but also address the emotional and social dimensions of TB.

Holistic Patient-Centered Care:
Patient-Centered Approach: Taking a holistic approach that considers the emotional wellbeing of the patient alongside medical treatment.
Counseling Services: Integrating mental health professionals into TB care teams.

- **Beyond the Diagnosis: Reintegration and Advocacy:**

Challenges: Life after TB treatment involves reintegration into society, often marked by residual stigma.

PostTreatment Support:
Follow-Up Care: Providing ongoing care to monitor physical and emotional wellbeing.
Advocacy Programs: Empowering individuals to become advocates for change, reducing stigma through their stories.

- **The Global Perspective: A Call for Solidarity**:

Challenges: TB affects individuals worldwide, and a global perspective is necessary for a unified approach.

International Collaborations:
Resource Sharing: Collaborating globally to share best practices, resources, and strategies.
Media's Role: Engaging media responsibly to portray TB accurately and challenge stereotypes.

Addressing the social and emotional aspects of TB requires a multidimensional approach involving individuals, communities, healthcare providers, and policymakers. By fostering understanding, empathy, and support, we can create a world where individuals affected by TB are not defined by their diagnosis but are embraced with compassion and solidarity.

CHAPTER 6: PREVENTION STRATEGIES

Prevention is an essential part of the global campaign to contain and eradicate tuberculosis (TB). The importance of vaccination programs and their effect on lowering the incidence of TB is highlighted in this chapter as it examines a variety of preventative interventions at both the individual and community levels.

Preventive Measures at Individual and Community Levels for Tuberculosis

Tuberculosis (TB) prevention involves a comprehensive approach that extends from individual practices to community-wide initiatives. This chapter delves into preventive measures at both the individual and community levels, emphasizing the importance of a collective effort in combating TB.

- **Individual-Level Preventive Measures:**

Infection Control Practices:

Respiratory Hygiene: Encouraging individuals to cover their mouth and nose when coughing or sneezing to prevent the spread of TB bacteria through respiratory droplets.

Ventilation: Promoting well-ventilated spaces, especially in crowded areas, to minimize the concentration of infectious particles.

Early Diagnosis and Treatment:

Timely Screening: Encouraging individuals with persistent coughs, unexplained weight loss, and other TB symptoms to seek prompt medical attention for diagnosis.

Adherence to Treatment: Emphasizing the importance of completing the full course of TB treatment to prevent the development of drug-resistant strains.

Education and Awareness:

Community Outreach: Conducting educational campaigns to raise awareness about TB, its symptoms, transmission, and preventive measures.

Stigma Reduction: Addressing misconceptions to reduce the stigma associated with TB and encourage early healthcare-seeking behavior.

- **Community-Level Preventive Measures:**

Contact Tracing:

Identification and screening: Identifying and screening individuals who have been in close contact with confirmed TB cases to detect latent infections early.

Prophylactic Treatment: Providing preventive therapy to individuals with latent TB infection to reduce the risk of progression to active disease.

Improved Living Conditions:

Overcrowding Reduction: Implementing measures to reduce overcrowding in households and community settings to lower the risk of TB transmission.

Sanitation and Nutrition Programs: Enhancing sanitation and nutrition programs to improve overall community health and resilience against TB.

Workplace Health Programs:

Occupational Screening: Implementing routine TB screening for individuals in high-risk occupations, such as healthcare workers and those working in congregate settings,

Workplace Education: Providing information about TB prevention and control in workplaces to protect employees and minimize transmission risks.

- **Innovative Technologies and Programs:**

New Diagnostic Technologies:

Point of Care Tests: Advancing the use of rapid diagnostic tools to detect TB early and facilitate prompt treatment initiation.

Mobile Health (mHealth): Utilizing mobile health technologies for TB awareness, education, and follow-up care, especially in remote or underserved areas.

Public-private Partnerships:

Collaborations for Accessible Diagnostics: Forging partnerships between the public and private sectors to ensure innovative diagnostic tools and preventive measures are accessible globally.

- **Behavioral Change Initiatives**:

Health Promotion Campaigns:

Lifestyle Education: Conducting campaigns to promote healthier lifestyles, emphasizing factors such as nutrition and exercise that contribute to overall community wellbeing and TB prevention.

Community Engagement:

Participatory Programs: Engaging communities in the design and implementation of TB prevention strategies to ensure cultural relevance and sustainability.

- **Global Collaboration for Prevention**:

International Cooperation:
Resource Sharing: Collaborating globally to share resources, knowledge, and best practices in TB prevention.
Research and Development Funding: Allocating funds for research and development of new prevention strategies, including vaccines and treatments.

Media and Advocacy:
Media Campaigns: Utilizing media platforms for public awareness campaigns to educate communities about preventive measures.
Advocacy Programs: Empowering individuals, communities, and organizations to advocate for increased funding and commitment to TB prevention on a global scale.

In conclusion, preventing tuberculosis requires a dual focus on individual behaviors and communitywide initiatives. By promoting awareness, fostering healthy practices, and leveraging technological advancements, societies can build a formidable defense against TB, working towards a world where the disease is effectively controlled and ultimately eliminated.

Exploring Vaccination Programs and Their Impact on Tuberculosis Prevention

Vaccination programs play a pivotal role in the prevention and control of infectious diseases, and tuberculosis (TB) is no exception. This section delves into the exploration of TB vaccination programs, focusing on the impact of the Bacillus Calmette-Guérin (BCG) vaccine and the ongoing efforts to develop more effective vaccines.

- **Bacillus Calmette-Guérin (BCG) Vaccine:**

Childhood Vaccination:
BCG is primarily administered in infancy, usually shortly after birth, in countries with a high prevalence of TB.

The vaccine is a live attenuated strain derived from Mycobacterium bovis, providing protection against severe forms of TB, especially in children.

Impact on Pediatric TB:

BCG vaccination has demonstrated significant efficacy in reducing the incidence of pediatric TB and preventing disseminated and severe forms of the disease.

The vaccine is credited with saving lives and reducing morbidity associated with childhood TB in the regions where it is implemented.

Variable Protection in Adults:

While BCG provides robust protection against certain forms of TB in children, its efficacy in preventing pulmonary TB in adults is variable and context-dependent.

Factors such as geography, strain variability, and exposure dynamics contribute to the variable effectiveness observed in adult populations.

- **Challenges and Opportunities:**

Limitations of BCG:

BCG does not offer consistent protection against pulmonary TB, the most common form of the disease in adults.

Its efficacy can wane over time, and there are limitations in regions with diverse circulating strains.

Ongoing Research and Development:

Researchers are actively exploring new strategies to enhance TB vaccine effectiveness, addressing the limitations of BCG.

Innovative approaches involve the development of subunit vaccines, viral vector vaccines, and adjuvanted formulations.

● Future Prospects in Vaccine Development:

Subunit Vaccines:

Subunit vaccines target specific antigens of Mycobacterium tuberculosis, potentially offering improved and more targeted protection.

Research is ongoing to identify optimal combinations of antigens that trigger strong and lasting immune responses.

Viral-Vectored Vaccines:

Viral vectored vaccines use modified viruses to carry TB antigens, enhancing the immune response.

Promising candidates are being evaluated for their safety and efficacy in clinical trials.

Adjuvanted Formulations:

Adjuvants are substances added to vaccines to enhance immune responses.

Adjuvanted TB vaccines are being explored to stimulate more robust and durable immunity.

- **Impact on TB Elimination**:

Herd Immunity and Transmission Reduction:
Effective TB vaccination not only protects individuals but can contribute to the reduction of TB transmission within communities.
Achieving high vaccination coverage is crucial for generating herd immunity and breaking the cycle of transmission.

Global Collaborations and Funding Initiatives:
The success of TB vaccination programs relies on international collaborations, funding support, and the commitment of governments and organizations to prioritize TB prevention.

- **Balancing Vaccination with Comprehensive TB Control**:

Integration with Other Prevention Strategies:

TB vaccination should be integrated into comprehensive TB control programs that include early diagnosis, treatment, and preventive therapy for latent TB infection.

Addressing Socio-Economic Factors:

Vaccination programs should be complemented by efforts to address socioeconomic factors that contribute to TB transmission, such as poverty, malnutrition, and inadequate healthcare access.

- **Public Perception and Communication**:

Public Awareness:

Effective communication is essential to ensuring public understanding of the benefits and limitations of TB vaccination.

Addressing vaccine hesitancy and providing accurate information contribute to successful vaccination programs.

Conclusion:

TB vaccination programs, particularly the BCG vaccine, have made significant strides in preventing severe forms of the disease, especially in children. Ongoing research and development efforts hold the promise of more effective vaccines that can contribute to the global goal of TB elimination. A multifaceted approach, integrating vaccination with other preventive strategies and addressing socioeconomic factors, is crucial for the success of TB control programs worldwide. Global collaborations, funding initiatives, and public awareness are key components in the journey towards a TB-free world.

CHAPTER 7: INNOVATIONS IN TB RESEARCH

Significant advancements in TB (tuberculosis) research have arisen in recent years, changing the way the disease is prevented, diagnosed, and treated. These discoveries offer hope for more effective and focused strategies to address this danger to global health.

Recent Breakthroughs in Tuberculosis Research

Tuberculosis (TB) research has witnessed significant breakthroughs in recent years, ushering in a new era of hope for effective prevention, diagnosis, and treatment. These breakthroughs reflect advancements across various facets of TB research, addressing challenges and providing innovative solutions.

- **Advancements in Diagnostics:**

Rapid Molecular Diagnostics:
Recent breakthroughs in molecular diagnostics, exemplified by technologies like GeneXpert, have revolutionized TB

diagnosis. These tools offer quick and accurate detection of TB and drug-resistant strains, even in resource-limited settings. This has significantly reduced the time between suspicion and the initiation of treatment.

Point of Care Testing:

Innovations in point-of-care testing have facilitated on-the-spot diagnosis, enabling faster and more accessible identification of TB cases. These rapid tests are particularly valuable in settings where timely access to diagnostic facilities is limited.

Artificial Intelligence (AI) Integration:

The integration of artificial intelligence algorithms into TB diagnostics, especially in the interpretation of chest X-rays, has enhanced accuracy and efficiency. AI-based tools aid in quicker and more reliable analysis, supporting healthcare professionals in making timely and informed decisions.

- **Therapeutic Breakthroughs:**

Novel Drugs:

The approval of novel drugs like bedaquiline and delamanid has expanded the arsenal of treatment options, particularly for multidrug-resistant TB. These drugs offer improved efficacy and tolerability, addressing a critical need in the management of drug-resistant strains.

Shortened Treatment Regimens:

Research into shortened treatment regimens aims to enhance patient adherence and reduce the overall duration of TB treatment. These innovations have the potential to improve treatment outcomes and reduce the burden on patients.

Host-directed Therapies:

The exploration of host-directed therapies represents a paradigm shift in TB treatment. Modulating the host immune response offers a new avenue for improving treatment effectiveness and addressing the complexities of TB pathogenesis.

- **Vaccine Development:**

Subunit Vaccines:

Advances in subunit vaccine development target specific TB antigens, aiming to provide more targeted and robust protection. These breakthroughs hold promise for the development of vaccines that elicit strong and durable immune responses.

Viral-Vectored Vaccines:
Research into viral-vectored TB vaccines is at the forefront of vaccine innovation. These vaccines leverage modified viruses to enhance immunogenicity, potentially leading to vaccines with improved efficacy.

- **Technological Innovations**:

Nanotechnology:
The integration of nanotechnology into TB research has yielded innovations in drug delivery and diagnostics. Nanoparticle drug delivery systems enhance the efficacy of antiTB medications, while nanodiagnostics provide sensitive and specific detection of TB biomarkers.

Digital Health Solutions:
Digital health solutions, including mobile health technologies, are transforming TB care. Digital contact tracing, remote monitoring of treatment adherence, and mobile health interventions contribute to more effective and patient-centered TB management.

- **Future Prospects**:

Precision Medicine:

The exploration of precision medicine in TB research involves understanding the genetic diversity of TB bacteria. This knowledge can inform personalized treatment strategies, optimizing therapeutic outcomes for individual patients.

Immunotherapies:

Immunotherapies, including cytokine therapies and T-cell immunotherapies, represent future prospects in TB treatment. These innovative approaches aim to modulate the immune response, potentially enhancing the body's ability to combat TB infection.

Global Collaborations and Data Sharing:

The formation of international consortia and initiatives for data sharing exemplifies a commitment to collaborative research. Such collaborations are essential for accelerating progress, especially in addressing global challenges like drug-resistant TB.

In conclusion, recent breakthroughs in TB research underscore the dynamic and evolving nature of efforts to combat this global health challenge. These innovations not only provide solutions to existing challenges but also pave the way for future advancements. As research continues to push boundaries, the hope is to translate these breakthroughs into tangible improvements in TB prevention, diagnosis, and treatment on a global scale.

Discussing Potential Future Developments in Tuberculosis Research

The landscape of tuberculosis (TB) research is dynamic, and potential future developments hold the promise of transformative advancements. Addressing challenges and pushing the boundaries of innovation is essential for achieving the global goal of TB control and elimination. Here, we explore potential future developments across various dimensions of TB research.

- **Precision Medicine in TB:**

Genomic Approaches:
Advancements in genomic medicine may lead to a deeper understanding of the genetic diversity of TB bacteria. This knowledge could pave the way for precision medicine approaches tailored to individual patients, optimizing treatment regimens based on the specific genetic characteristics of the infecting strain.

Pharmacogenomics:
The integration of pharmacogenomic approaches in TB research holds the potential to personalize drug regimens based on an individual's genetic profile. Understanding how an individual's genetic makeup influences their response to TB medications could enhance treatment outcomes and reduce the risk of adverse effects.

- **Immunotherapies**:

Cytokine Therapies:
Future developments may involve the use of cytokine therapies to modulate the immune response in TB. Targeted administration of specific cytokines could enhance the host's ability to control TB infection, leading to more effective and nuanced treatment strategies.

T-CELL Immunotherapies:
Research into T-cell immunotherapies as adjunctive treatments for TB aims to harness the power of the immune system. By boosting T-cell responses, these therapies could contribute to better outcomes, especially in cases of drug-resistant TB.

- Nanotechnology in TB Management:

Nanoparticle Drug Delivery:
Continued advancements in nanotechnology may lead to the development of more sophisticated nanoparticle drug delivery systems. These systems could improve the targeted delivery of antiTB medications, enhancing efficacy while minimizing side effects.

Nanodiagnostics:
The refinement of nanodiagnostics holds the potential for even more sensitive and specific detection of TB biomarkers. Nanoscale technologies could revolutionize diagnostic accuracy, especially in settings where traditional diagnostic methods may be limited.

- Public Health Innovations:

Integrated Care Platforms:
Future developments may see the integration of TB care into broader healthcare platforms. Comprehensive, integrated care could address not only the medical aspects of TB but also social determinants and comorbidities, leading to more holistic patient outcomes.

Community-based Interventions:
Expanding community-based interventions with the use of technology and community health workers could enhance outreach and engagement. Leveraging digital health solutions, including mobile health (mHealth), may play a significant role in ensuring effective community-based TB programs.

- **Global Collaborations and Data Sharing**:

International Consortia:
The formation of international consortia for collaborative TB research may deepen global collaboration. Sharing expertise, resources, and data on a global scale can accelerate progress, particularly in addressing challenges like emerging drug-resistant strains.

Data Sharing Initiatives:
Strengthening data-sharing initiatives is crucial for advancing TB research. Improved sharing of research findings, clinical data, and genomic information can foster a more comprehensive and collaborative approach to understanding and combating TB.

- **Challenges and Ethical Considerations**:

Antimicrobial Resistance:

Future developments must address the challenge of emerging drug-resistant TB strains. Research initiatives should focus on strategies to prevent the further spread of resistance and develop innovative treatments.

Access to Innovations:

Ensuring equitable access to new diagnostic tools, drugs, and vaccines remains a critical consideration. Future developments should prioritize strategies to make innovative TB solutions affordable and accessible globally.

As TB research continues to evolve, these potential future developments represent exciting possibilities for shaping a more effective, patient-centered, and globally collaborative approach to TB prevention, diagnosis, and treatment. The success of these endeavors will rely on sustained research efforts, international collaboration, and a commitment to addressing the multifaceted challenges posed by TB.

CHAPTER 8: STIGMA AND TB

In addition to being a medical problem, tuberculosis (TB) also presents a social and cultural difficulty. The stigma attached to TB has wide-ranging effects on people, families, and entire communities. This chapter explores the intricate problem of TB stigma in an effort to increase knowledge, foster comprehension, and push for significant change.

Addressing the Stigma Associated with Tuberculosis

Tuberculosis (TB) remains not only a medical challenge but also a social one, with a history of stigma and discrimination attached to it. Addressing the stigma associated with TB is essential for promoting early diagnosis, treatment adherence, and the overall well-being of individuals and communities. This section explores strategies and initiatives aimed at tackling TB-related stigma.

- **Education and Awareness Campaigns:**

Dispelling Myths and Misinformation:

Community Outreach: Conducting educational campaigns at the community level to dispel myths and misconceptions about TB. This involves providing accurate information about the causes, transmission, and curability of the disease.

School Programs: Integrating TB education into school curricula to reach younger generations and foster a culture of understanding and empathy.

Media Engagement:

Media Campaigns: Leveraging various media channels to disseminate accurate information about TB. This includes TV and radio advertisements, documentaries, and social media campaigns that highlight stories of recovery and resilience.

Collaboration with Influencers: Collaborating with social media influencers and celebrities to amplify awareness and reduce stigma.

- **Empowering Affected Communities**:

Support Groups:

Establishment of Support Groups: Creating safe spaces for individuals affected by TB to share their experiences, challenges, and successes. Support groups provide emotional support, reduce isolation, and foster a sense of community.

Community-based Programs: Engaging local communities in TB awareness programs to empower them to challenge stigma at the grassroots level.

Involvement of Survivors:

Advocacy by Survivors: Encouraging individuals who have successfully completed TB treatment to become advocates. Their stories can serve as powerful testimonials, challenging stereotypes and promoting understanding.

- **Advocacy and Policy Initiatives**:

Legal Protections:

Advocacy for Legal Protections: Advocating for legal measures that protect individuals from discrimination based on their TB status. This includes workplace protections and anti-discrimination laws.

Policy Integration: Ensuring that anti-stigma initiatives are integrated into national and global TB control policies. This involves addressing social determinants of TB, such as poverty and lack of education.

- **Changing Narratives**:

Humanizing Stories:

Personal Testimonies: Sharing personal stories of individuals living with TB to humanize the experience. These narratives counter stigmatizing stereotypes and provide a face to the disease.

Cultural Sensitivity: Tailoring awareness campaigns to specific cultural contexts to ensure relevance and resonance.

Healthcare Provider Sensitization:

Training Programs: Implementing training programs for healthcare providers to sensitize them to the impact of stigma. This includes equipping them with communication skills to address stigma in clinical settings.

Patient-centered Care: Promoting patient-centered care that respects the dignity and rights of individuals affected by TB.

- **Collaboration and Partnerships**:

Multi-Sectoral Collaboration:

Engaging Stakeholders: Collaborating with governmental and non-governmental organizations, community leaders, and the private sector to create a united front against TB stigma.

Cross-Sectoral Programs: Implementing programs that address social determinants of TB, such as poverty and lack of education, through collaborations across different sectors.

International Collaboration:

Global Campaigns: Participating in and supporting global campaigns to eliminate TB stigma. Emphasizing the interconnectedness of efforts is crucial in a world with increasing population mobility.

- **The Role of Media and Technology**:

Positive Messaging:

Media Campaigns: Collaborating with media outlets to create positive and accurate portrayals of TB. This involves emphasizing recovery stories and showcasing the resilience of individuals affected by TB.

Social Media Activism: Utilizing social media platforms for grassroots activism, fostering a sense of solidarity, and breaking down barriers by promoting positive TB-related content.

- **Evaluation and Continuous Improvement:**

Monitoring and Evaluation:

Assessment of Interventions: Regularly assessing the impact of antistigma interventions through monitoring and evaluation. This involves gathering feedback from communities and individuals to understand the effectiveness of strategies.

Adapting Approaches: Being flexible and adaptive in approaches based on the evolving needs and challenges related to TB stigma.

Addressing the stigma associated with tuberculosis is a multifaceted task that requires collaboration, education, and a commitment to changing societal attitudes. By combining community empowerment, policy advocacy, and positive storytelling, it is possible to reduce stigma and create an environment where individuals affected by TB can seek help without fear of discrimination. This chapter advocates for sustained efforts to eliminate TB stigma, emphasizing the importance of a holistic and people-centered approach.

Advocating for Awareness and Understanding

Advocating for awareness and understanding is a pivotal strategy in addressing complex issues such as diseases, particularly those accompanied by stigma, misinformation, and social challenges. This section explores the importance of advocacy in promoting awareness and understanding, with a focus on tuberculosis (TB).

- **The Significance of Advocacy:**

Shaping Perceptions:

Countering Misinformation: Advocacy plays a crucial role in countering misinformation about TB. By providing accurate information, advocates contribute to shaping public perceptions and dispelling myths surrounding the disease.

Challenging Stigma: Advocacy initiatives challenge the stigma associated with TB, creating an environment where individuals affected by the disease are understood, supported, and treated with dignity.

Mobilizing Support:

Community Engagement: Advocacy mobilizes communities by engaging individuals, local leaders, and organizations. This collective mobilization is essential for building a supportive network and fostering a sense of shared responsibility.

Policy Influence: Advocacy can influence policy decisions by highlighting the importance of TB awareness in national and global health agendas. This includes advocating for resources, research, and equitable access to healthcare.

- **Strategies for Advocacy:**

Media Campaigns:

Public Service Announcements: Advocacy through media campaigns, including public service announcements on television, radio, and social media, helps disseminate accurate information about TB.

Documentaries and Interviews: Feature documentaries and interviews with experts and individuals affected by TB contribute to a more nuanced and human understanding of the disease.

Grassroots Initiatives:

Community Workshops: Organizing workshops at the community level to educate individuals about TB, its transmission, treatment, and the importance of early diagnosis.

Storytelling and Art: Using storytelling, art, and cultural activities to convey messages that resonate with diverse audiences, breaking down barriers and fostering empathy.

Advocacy Networks:

Collaborative Partnerships: Building collaborative networks with nongovernmental organizations, healthcare providers, and affected communities to amplify advocacy efforts.

Global Alliances: Participating in global alliances and coalitions dedicated to TB advocacy to leverage collective influence and share best practices.

- **Tailoring Messages for Impact:**

Targeted Messaging:

Addressing Diverse Audiences: Advocacy messages should be tailored to address the diverse needs of different populations, considering cultural, linguistic, and socioeconomic factors.

Emphasizing Shared Responsibility: Messages should emphasize that TB is a shared responsibility, encouraging communities to play an active role in prevention, treatment, and support.

Humanizing the Impact:

Personal Stories: Sharing personal stories of individuals affected by TB humanizes the impact of the disease, fostering empathy and understanding.

Highlighting Success Stories: Showcasing success stories of communities that have effectively tackled TB-related challenges demonstrates the positive impact of awareness and understanding.

- **Education as a Tool for Advocacy**:

School Programs:

Incorporating TB Education: Advocacy efforts can extend to school programs, incorporating TB education into curricula to inform and empower future generations.

Youth Engagement: engaging youth in advocacy initiatives, empowering them as advocates for TB awareness within their communities.

Healthcare Provider Training:

Sensitizing Healthcare Providers: Advocacy can include training programs for healthcare providers, ensuring they have the knowledge and skills to communicate effectively with patients and address TB-related stigma.

- **Advocacy Metrics and Evaluation**:

Measuring Impact:

Tracking Awareness Levels: Utilizing metrics to measure changes in awareness levels within communities over time.

Evaluating Policy Impact: Assessing the impact of advocacy efforts on policy changes and resource allocation for TB prevention and treatment.

Advocating for awareness and understanding is a catalyst for positive change in the context of complex health issues like tuberculosis. By strategically employing media campaigns, grassroots initiatives, and targeted education, advocates can challenge stigma, dispel misinformation, and create a global environment where TB is understood, prevented, and effectively managed. The ongoing commitment to advocacy ensures that awareness efforts continue to evolve, adapt, and resonate with diverse audiences, ultimately contributing to a world where TB is not only treatable but also destigmatized and preventable.

CHAPTER 9: PUBLIC HEALTH POLICIES AND TB CONTROL

A complete and effective set of control and preventative measures is needed for tuberculosis (TB), which continues to be a problem for worldwide public health. This chapter examines TB control public health initiatives on a national and worldwide level. It explores the accomplishments made and the difficulties encountered and suggests adjustments to strengthen the battle against TB.

Examining National and International Policies to Control Tuberculosis

Tuberculosis (TB) remains a significant global health challenge, necessitating robust national and international policies for effective control and prevention. This examination seeks to assess the strengths, challenges, and proposed improvements in existing policies aimed at combating TB at both the national and international levels.

- **National Policies:**

Overview:

National Tuberculosis Control Programs (NTPs): Many countries have established NTPs that outline strategies for TB prevention, diagnosis, and treatment.

Guidelines and Protocols: National policies often include guidelines and protocols for TB diagnosis, treatment, and control measures.

Successes:

Diagnostic Advancements: Policies emphasizing the adoption of advanced diagnostic tools, such as GeneXpert, have led to quicker and more accurate TB diagnosis.

Treatment Standardization: Standardized treatment protocols, such as Directly Observed Treatment, and Short Course (DOTS), have contributed to improved treatment outcomes.

Challenges:

Fragmented Healthcare Systems: Fragmentation within healthcare systems can lead to challenges in the seamless implementation of TB control policies.

Access Disparities: Disparities in access to TB services, particularly in rural and marginalized communities, can result in delayed diagnosis and treatment.

Proposed Improvements:

Integrated Healthcare: Strengthening integration between TB control programs and general healthcare services for a more cohesive approach.

Community Engagement: Enhancing community engagement to bridge access gaps, promote awareness, and facilitate education at the grassroots level.

- **International Policies:**

Global Strategies:

End TB Strategy: The World Health Organization's (WHO) End TB Strategy outlines global targets for TB control, emphasizing prevention, treatment, and research.

Global Fund Initiatives: International collaborations, such as those supported by the Global Fund, contribute funding to bolster TB control efforts.

Successes:

Global Incidence Reduction: International efforts have contributed to a decline in TB incidence globally.

Increased Funding: Mobilization of international resources has enabled the scaling up of TB prevention and treatment programs.

Challenges:

Cross-Border Issues: TB control faces challenges in regions with porous borders and significant population movement.

Funding Gaps: Despite progress, funding gaps persist, hindering the implementation of comprehensive TB control measures.

Proposed Improvements:

Cross-Border Collaboration: Strengthening collaboration between countries to address cross-border challenges and ensure coordinated TB control efforts.

Innovative Financing Models: Exploring innovative financing models to address funding gaps and sustain long-term TB control initiatives.

- **Policy Challenges in Addressing Drug-Resistant TB:**

Multidrug-resistant TB (MDR TB):

Treatment Challenges: MDR TB poses significant challenges, requiring prolonged and complex drug regimens.

Limited Access to Diagnosis: Challenges in accessing accurate and timely diagnostics for MDR TB contribute to delayed treatment initiation.

Proposed Improvements:

Streamlined Drug Regimens: Research and development of more streamlined and effective drug regimens for MDR TB.

Improved Diagnostic Technologies: Investment in research for improved and accessible diagnostic technologies for drug-resistant TB.

- **Technological Integration in TB Control:**

Digital Health Solutions:

Mobile Health (mHealth): Integration of mHealth technologies for patient education, treatment adherence monitoring, and data reporting.

Digital Contact Tracing: Utilizing digital tools for effective contact tracing, especially in densely populated areas.

Challenges:

Technological Disparities: Unequal access to technology poses challenges, particularly in low-resource settings.

Data Security Concerns: Ensuring the security and privacy of patient data in digital health systems.

Proposed Improvements:

Capacity Building: Investing in capacity building to ensure that healthcare providers and communities are equipped to utilize digital health tools effectively.

International Collaboration on Standards: Collaborating on international standards for data security and interoperability in digital health solutions.

The examination of national and international policies to control tuberculosis reveals both successes and challenges. Strengthening these policies requires a concerted effort to address gaps in healthcare systems, promote international collaboration, secure sustainable funding, and leverage technological advancements. By implementing the proposed improvements and fostering a holistic, multifaceted approach, nations and the global community can move closer to the ultimate goal of eliminating tuberculosis and achieving a world free from the burdens of this infectious disease.

Discussing Challenges and Proposing Improvements in TB Control Policies

- **National Policies:**

Challenges:

Fragmentation: Fragmentation within healthcare systems can impede the seamless implementation of TB control policies. Streamlining services and enhancing coordination between different healthcare entities is critical.

Access Disparities: Rural and marginalized populations often face difficulties in accessing TB services, leading to delayed diagnosis and treatment. Tailoring policies to address geographical and socioeconomic disparities is essential.

Proposed Improvements:

Integrated Healthcare: Strengthening integration between TB control programs and general healthcare services to provide a more cohesive and patient-centered approach.

Community Engagement: Implementing strategies to engage communities actively, promote awareness, and ensure that healthcare services are accessible to all.

- **International Policies:**

Challenges:

Cross-Border Issues: TB control faces challenges in regions with porous borders and significant population movement. Enhancing international collaboration is crucial for addressing these cross-border challenges.

Funding Gaps: Despite progress, funding gaps persist, hindering the implementation of comprehensive TB control measures globally. Exploring innovative financing models and strengthening financial commitments are necessary.

Proposed Improvements:

Cross-Border Collaboration: Strengthening collaboration between countries to address cross-border issues and ensure a coordinated, global response to TB.

Innovative Financing Models: Exploring and implementing innovative financing models, such as public-private partnerships and impact investing, to bridge funding gaps and sustain long-term TB control initiatives.

- **Drug-resistant TB:**

Challenges:

Treatment Complexity: Multidrug-resistant TB (MDR TB) poses significant challenges due to the complexity of treatment regimens. Developing more streamlined and patient-friendly drug regimens is imperative.

Limited Access to Diagnosis: Challenges in accessing accurate and timely diagnostics for drug-resistant TB contribute to delayed treatment initiation. Improving diagnostic technologies and ensuring their accessibility are critical.

Proposed Improvements:

Streamlined Drug Regimens: Research and development of more patient-friendly and effective drug regimens for MDR TB, reducing the burden on patients.

Improved Diagnostic Technologies: Investment in research to develop and deploy improved and accessible diagnostic technologies for drug-resistant TB.

- **Technological Integration:**

Challenges:

Technological Disparities: Unequal access to technology poses challenges, particularly in low-resource settings. Efforts should be made to bridge these disparities and ensure widespread access.

Data Security Concerns: Ensuring the security and privacy of patient data in digital health systems is a paramount concern. Establishing robust standards and protocols is essential.

Proposed Improvements:

Capacity Building: Investing in capacity building to ensure that healthcare providers and communities are equipped to utilize digital health tools effectively.

International Collaboration on Standards: Collaborating on international standards for data security and interoperability in digital health solutions to address concerns and ensure ethical use of technology.

The challenges in TB control policies are diverse and require multifaceted solutions. Proposing improvements involves addressing system-level issues, enhancing collaboration, and embracing innovation. National and international policymakers, healthcare professionals, and communities must work together to implement these improvements. By doing so, we can overcome the challenges, fortify TB control policies, and move closer to achieving the ultimate goal of eliminating tuberculosis globally.

CHAPTER 10: THE ROLE OF COMMUNITIES

The battle against tuberculosis (TB) requires a collective effort, with communities playing a pivotal role in prevention, care, and support. This chapter delves into the indispensable role communities play in the fight against TB, emphasizing the importance of community engagement and showcasing successful community-based initiatives

Exploring the Crucial Role Communities Play in TB Prevention and Care

Tuberculosis (TB) is not merely a medical challenge; it is a complex social issue that requires a community-driven approach for effective prevention and care. This exploration delves into the crucial role communities play in the fight against TB, highlighting their impact on prevention, early detection, treatment adherence, and overall support for individuals affected by the disease.

- **Early Detection through Community Vigilance:**

Vigilant Community Members:

Communities act as the first line of defense in detecting TB cases. Vigilant community members, equipped with basic health knowledge, can recognize symptoms early on.

Heightened awareness within communities leads to early medical consultation, facilitating prompt diagnosis and treatment initiation.

Health Literacy Empowerment:

Empowering communities with health literacy is instrumental. Understanding the symptoms, modes of transmission, and importance of seeking medical help equips individuals to take proactive measures.

Health education programs within communities contribute to a population that is informed and alert to the signs of TB.

- **Treatment Adherence and Support:**

Community Support Networks:

Building support networks within communities is crucial for individuals undergoing TB treatment. Emotional and practical support from peers fosters a sense of community and reduces the risk of treatment abandonment.

Supportive environments within communities contribute to a higher likelihood of treatment success.

Addressing Stigma:

TB-related stigma is a significant barrier to care. Communities play a vital role in addressing and dismantling this stigma.

Open conversations, educational initiatives, and community-led advocacy help dispel misconceptions and create a more supportive atmosphere for those affected by TB.

- **Successful Community-Based Initiatives:**

Community Health Workers (CHWs):

Training and Empowerment: Community health workers serve as essential bridges between healthcare systems and communities. Training and empowering them as TB educators and advocates enhances their effectiveness.

Home-Based Care: CHWs engaged in home-based care initiatives ensure that patients receive personalized attention, contributing to improved treatment outcomes.

TB Support Groups:

Peer Support: Support groups provide a platform for individuals affected by TB to share experiences, challenges, and successes. Peer support is invaluable in navigating the emotional and social dimensions of TB.

Community-Led Advocacy: Engaging support groups in advocacy efforts amplifies community voices, driving positive changes in TB policies and services.

Awareness Campaigns:

Local Media Engagement: Utilizing local media channels for targeted awareness campaigns ensures that information reaches diverse community segments.

Cultural Sensitivity: Awareness materials tailored to reflect cultural contexts are more likely to resonate, fostering a deeper understanding of TB within the community.

- **Challenges in Community Involvement:**

Limited Resources:

Financial Constraints: Many communities, especially in resource-limited settings, face financial constraints in implementing and sustaining community-based initiatives.

Infrastructure Gaps: Lack of proper infrastructure can hinder the effectiveness of community-led initiatives, impacting the reach and impact of TB awareness and support programs.

Stigma and Discrimination:

Addressing Deep-Rooted Stigma: Overcoming deep-rooted societal stigma requires persistent efforts in education, advocacy, and fostering empathy within communities.

Ensuring Inclusivity: Community initiatives must be designed to be inclusive, avoiding the unintentional perpetuation of stigma against individuals affected by TB.

- **Recommendations for Strengthening Community Engagement:**

Capacity Building:

Training Programs: Implementing training programs for community health workers and volunteers to enhance their knowledge and skills in TB prevention, care, and advocacy.

Resource Mobilization: Facilitating access to resources, including financial support and technological tools, to strengthen community-led initiatives.

Collaboration with Healthcare Providers:

Partnerships: Facilitating partnerships between communities and healthcare providers ensures a continuum of care and support for individuals affected by TB.

Health Worker Sensitization: Conducting sensitization programs for healthcare providers to enhance their understanding of the role communities play and foster collaboration.

Communities are not passive recipients but active contributors to the fight against TB. Their engagement is essential for building resilient healthcare systems. Recognizing and strengthening the role of communities in TB prevention and care is fundamental to achieving sustainable progress in the global effort to eliminate tuberculosis. This exploration underscores the significance of community involvement, showcases successful initiatives, and outlines recommendations for further enhancing community participation in the journey toward a TB-free world.

Showcasing Successful Community-Based Initiatives in TB Prevention and Care

Communities are integral partners in the global effort to combat tuberculosis (TB). Successful community-based initiatives not only contribute to the prevention and early detection of TB but also play a crucial role in providing support and reducing stigma for those affected. This showcase highlights exemplary initiatives that demonstrate the power of community engagement in the fight against TB.

- **Community Health Workers (CHWs) Empowerment**:

Initiative Overview:

Training and Education: In several communities, initiatives have been implemented to empower local individuals as community health workers. These CHWs undergo comprehensive training on TB prevention, symptoms, and treatment adherence.

Home-Based Education and Support: Trained CHWs visit homes to educate families about TB, conduct screenings, and provide ongoing support to individuals undergoing treatment.

Impact:

Increased Awareness: This initiative has significantly increased awareness about TB within communities, leading to early detection and improved health-seeking behavior.

Enhanced Treatment Adherence: Through personalized support, CHWs have contributed to higher rates of treatment adherence, reducing the risk of treatment abandonment.

- **TB Support Groups**:

Initiative Overview:

Establishment of Support Networks: TB support groups have been formed to create a sense of community among individuals affected by TB. These groups provide a platform for sharing experiences, offering emotional support, and advocating for better services.

Community-Led Advocacy: Some support groups actively engage in advocacy efforts, collaborating with healthcare organizations and policymakers to address gaps in TB services.

Impact:

Emotional Support: Support groups have proven to be invaluable in addressing the emotional aspects of TB, reducing isolation, and fostering a sense of belonging.

Advocacy Success Stories: Communities engaged in advocacy efforts have contributed to policy changes, leading to improved TB services and reduced stigma.

- **Mobile Health (mHealth) Solutions:**

Initiative Overview:

Utilization of Mobile Applications: Some communities have embraced mobile health solutions to disseminate TB information, provide virtual support, and facilitate treatment adherence.

Text Messaging for Reminders: Mobile applications send reminders for medication adherence, reducing the risk of missed doses.

Impact:

Widespread Information Dissemination: Mobile health applications have been effective in reaching diverse populations, especially in areas with limited access to traditional healthcare.

Improved Adherence: Text reminders and virtual support contribute to improved treatment adherence, ensuring that individuals complete their prescribed courses.

- **CommunityLed Awareness Campaigns:**

Initiative Overview:

Local Media Engagement: Communities have successfully used local media channels, including radio and community newsletters, to conduct targeted awareness campaigns.

Cultural Sensitivity: Awareness materials are tailored to reflect cultural contexts, ensuring that the information is relatable and resonant.

Impact:

Increased Knowledge: These initiatives have led to increased knowledge about TB symptoms, prevention, and treatment options within communities.

Reduced Stigma: By addressing misconceptions and fostering understanding, community-led campaigns contribute to reducing TB-related stigma.

- **Community-Based Screening Programs:**

Initiative Overview:

Screenings: Some communities have implemented door-to-door door-to-door programs where trained volunteers conduct screenings within neighborhoods.

Collaboration with Healthcare Providers: Positive cases are seamlessly linked with healthcare providers for further diagnosis and treatment.

Impact:

Early Detection: Community-based screening programs have led to the early detection of TB cases, allowing for prompt medical intervention.

Improved Access to Healthcare: By collaborating with healthcare providers, these initiatives bridge the gap between communities and formal healthcare systems.

These showcased community-based initiatives demonstrate the transformative impact of community engagement in TB prevention and care. From empowered community health workers to advocacy-driven support groups and innovative mHealth solutions, communities are actively contributing to the global goal of eliminating tuberculosis. By learning from these successes, adapting strategies to local contexts, and fostering collaborative partnerships, communities worldwide can continue to play a crucial role in creating a TB-free future.

CHAPTER 11: GLOBAL PARTNERSHIPS IN TB ERADICATION

The battle against tuberculosis (TB) is an international issue that necessitates unprecedented levels of cooperation. This chapter explores the value of international collaboration in tackling the many problems that this infectious illness presents. It focuses on the vital role that international cooperation plays in the eradication of TB.

Discussing Collaborative Efforts on a Global Scale to Combat Tuberculosis (TB)

Tuberculosis (TB) is a global health challenge that necessitates united efforts on an international scale. This chapter delves into the collaborative initiatives and partnerships that have been instrumental in the fight against TB, emphasizing the significance of a coordinated global response to tackle this infectious disease.

- **Global Health Organizations:**

World Health Organization (WHO):

The WHO plays a central role in setting global standards and guidelines for TB prevention, diagnosis, and treatment.

It facilitates the exchange of information, best practices, and resources among member countries to strengthen their TB programs.

The Global Fund:

As a major financial contributor, the Global Fund supports TB programs worldwide, providing funding for essential interventions such as diagnosis, treatment, and prevention.

It operates as a partnership between governments, civil society, and the private sector, emphasizing collaboration in addressing the global TB burden.

- **Multilateral Initiatives:**

Stop TB Partnership:

The Stop TB Partnership serves as a collaborative platform bringing together governments, nongovernmental organizations (NGOs), and private sector entities.

Its focus is on accelerating progress toward the goals outlined in the WHO's End TB Strategy.

UNITAID:

UNITAID contributes to global TB efforts by facilitating access to innovative tools, diagnostics, and treatments.

By leveraging partnerships and investments, UNITAID addresses critical gaps in TB care and control.

• The Importance of International Cooperation:

Data Sharing and Surveillance:
Global collaboration enables the sharing of epidemiological data, contributing to a comprehensive understanding of TB trends.

Surveillance networks foster early detection of outbreaks and the monitoring of drug resistance patterns on a global scale.

Research and Development:
Collaborative research consortia pool resources and expertise to develop new diagnostics, drugs, and vaccines.

International cooperation in research accelerates progress and ensures that advancements are accessible to diverse populations.

Capacity Building:

Global training initiatives empower healthcare professionals with the knowledge and skills necessary for effective TB prevention, diagnosis, and treatment.

Educational exchanges facilitate the sharing of expertise, promoting a more robust global healthcare workforce.

- **Challenges in Global Partnerships:**

Funding Gaps:

Persistent funding gaps hinder the implementation of comprehensive TB programs globally.

Sustainable financing models and innovative funding mechanisms are essential for addressing these gaps.

Political Commitment:

Achieving alignment between national policies and global strategies requires sustained political commitment.

Global advocacy efforts are necessary to keep TB high on political agendas and mobilize resources.

- **Success Stories in Global Cooperation:**

The End TB Strategy:

Global partnerships have contributed to a reduction in TB incidence, showcasing progress toward the ambitious targets set by the End TB Strategy.

Advances in diagnostics and treatment protocols reflect the impact of collaborative efforts.

Addressing Drug-Resistant TB:

International collaboration in drug development has shown promise in addressing drug-resistant TB.

Streamlined treatment protocols have been developed through global partnerships, enhancing patient outcomes.

- **Future Directions in Global TB Eradication:**

Strengthening Health Systems:

Prioritizing healthcare infrastructure development in TB endemic regions is crucial.

Investments in human resource development will enhance the capacity of local healthcare systems.

Advocacy and Awareness:

Global campaigns and advocacy efforts are essential for raising awareness about TB and reducing stigma.

Inclusive communication strategies will ensure that diverse populations are reached effectively.

Collaborative efforts on a global scale are indispensable in the battle against TB. This chapter underscores the vital role played by global health organizations, multilateral initiatives, and international cooperation. While challenges persist, the success stories exemplify the impact of united efforts. Looking ahead, sustaining political commitment, addressing funding gaps, and fostering inclusive collaborations are pivotal for achieving the ultimate goal of eradicating TB worldwide. Through shared responsibility and collective action, the global community can make significant strides toward a TB-free future.

Highlighting the Importance of International Cooperation in Combating Tuberculosis (TB)

Tuberculosis (TB) poses a significant global health challenge that transcends national borders. Highlighting the importance of international cooperation is crucial for addressing the complex, interconnected issues associated with TB. This section underscores the reasons why collaboration on an international scale is indispensable in the fight against TB.

- **Global Nature of TB:**

Transboundary Threat:

TB does not adhere to geopolitical boundaries. It spreads across borders, affecting people irrespective of nationality, ethnicity, or socioeconomic status.

International cooperation is essential to creating a unified front against a disease that respects no borders.

- **Sharing Resources and Expertise:**

Resource Mobilization:

TBendemic regions often face resource constraints, hindering their ability to implement comprehensive prevention and treatment programs.

International cooperation allows for the pooling of financial resources, ensuring that affected regions receive the necessary support to strengthen their healthcare systems.

Expertise Exchange:

Collaborative efforts enable the exchange of knowledge, skills, and best practices among countries with varying levels of experience in managing TB.

Experienced nations can provide guidance and mentorship to regions facing challenges in implementing effective TB control strategies.

- **Research and Development:**

Accelerating Progress:
International collaboration in research accelerates the development of new diagnostics, drugs, and vaccines.

Collective efforts ensure that advancements in TB science are shared globally, speeding up progress and improving outcomes for patients worldwide.

Addressing Drug-Resistant TB:
Drug-resistant TB poses a formidable challenge that requires innovative solutions.

Global partnerships in research and development aim to discover and implement new treatment regimens for drug-resistant TB, benefiting individuals in all corners of the world.

- **Strengthening Health Systems:**

Capacity Building:
Many TBendemic regions lack the necessary infrastructure and skilled healthcare workforce to effectively combat the disease.

International cooperation focuses on capacity building and providing training and resources to strengthen local health systems.

Sustainable Solutions:
Collaborative efforts prioritize the development of sustainable healthcare solutions that are tailored to the specific needs of diverse communities.

By working together, nations can create resilient health systems capable of withstanding the challenges posed by TB.

- **Addressing Social Determinants:**

Socioeconomic Factors:
TB is closely linked to social determinants such as poverty, inadequate housing, and a lack of education.

International cooperation recognizes the need to address these broader social issues, fostering a holistic approach to TB prevention and care.

- **Advocacy and Awareness:**

Global Advocacy:

A unified international front amplifies advocacy efforts, ensuring that TB remains a priority on the global health agenda.

Advocacy initiatives aim to reduce stigma, increase public awareness, and mobilize support for TB control programs.

Inclusive Communication:

Communication strategies that are culturally sensitive and inclusive reach diverse populations more effectively.

International cooperation in communication ensures that information about TB is disseminated in a manner that is accessible and relatable to people worldwide.

- **Global Health Security:**

Preventing Global Health Crises:

TB, if left uncontrolled, has the potential to escalate into a global health crisis.

International cooperation in TB control is not only about improving the health of individual nations but also about safeguarding global health security.

In conclusion, the importance of international cooperation in combating TB cannot be overstated. The interconnectedness of global health demands collaborative efforts that transcend borders. By sharing resources, expertise, and a collective commitment to addressing the social determinants of TB, the international community can make significant strides toward eliminating this infectious disease. Through united and sustained action, the vision of a world free from the burden of tuberculosis can be realized.

CONCLUSION: A BRIGHTER FUTURE WITHOUT TB

In concluding this exploration of tuberculosis (TB) and the global efforts to combat it, we reflect on key insights gleaned from the various chapters. The journey through the historical perspective, global impact, challenges, and collaborative initiatives has provided a comprehensive understanding of the complexities surrounding TB. As we look to the future, it is evident that concerted international cooperation is paramount in our quest for a world free from the burden of tuberculosis.

- **Historical Perspective and Global Impact:**

Understanding the Past: Tracing the history of TB has illuminated its profound impact on societies across centuries. From historical accounts to modern challenges, TB has left an indelible mark on human history.

Global Impact: TB's reach knows no borders. It is a global health challenge that requires a united response to tackle its multifaceted dimensions.

- **Collaborative Efforts and Global Partnerships:**

International Cooperation: The importance of international cooperation cannot be overstated. Global health organizations, multilateral initiatives, and collaborative efforts are essential in addressing the global nature of TB.

Sharing Resources: Through the sharing of resources, expertise, and a commitment to research and development, nations can collectively work towards more effective prevention, diagnosis, and treatment strategies.

- **Challenges and Opportunities:**

Funding and Political Commitment: The challenges of funding gaps and political commitment persist, requiring sustained efforts to bridge these gaps.

Opportunities for Innovation: Despite challenges, there are promising opportunities for innovation in diagnostics, drugs, and vaccines, providing hope for more effective TB control in the future.

A Call to Action

Individual and Collective Responsibility: The fight against TB is not just the responsibility of governments and healthcare institutions. It is a collective endeavor that requires the involvement of individuals, communities, and the private sector.

Advocacy and Awareness: Advocacy and raising awareness play a crucial role in reducing stigma, increasing public understanding, and mobilizing support for TB control programs.

A Brighter Future Without TB

Sustainable Solutions: By prioritizing sustainable healthcare solutions and addressing social determinants, we pave the way for a brighter future without TB.

Resilient Health Systems: Strengthening health systems globally ensures that communities are better equipped to face health challenges, including TB.

Encouragement for Readers

As readers, you are not just passive observers but potential change makers. Your understanding, awareness, and advocacy can contribute to the global movement to conquer tuberculosis. Embrace the role of advocates, champions, and informed citizens in the quest for a world where TB is but a historical footnote.

In conclusion, the journey to a brighter future without TB is one of shared responsibility and collective action. By building on the lessons of the past, embracing innovation, and fostering a global community committed to health equity, we can envision a world where TB is no longer a threat. Let us be part of this movement, working together towards a future where the pages of history tell the story of a world that conquered tuberculosis.